Aromatherapy

Essential Oils for Harmony and Health

Second Edition
Revised and Updated

Deanne Tenney

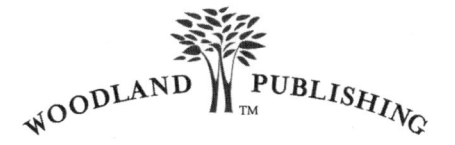

WOODLAND PUBLISHING

Copyright © 2007 by Deanne Tenney

All rights reserved. No part of this publication may be reproduced, stored in a retrieval system, or transmitted in any form without the prior written permission of the copyright owner.

For permissions, ordering information, or bulk quantity discounts, contact:
Woodland Publishing, 448 East 800 North, Orem, Utah 84097

Visit our Web site: www.woodlandpublishing.com
Toll-free number: (800) 777-2665

The information in this book is for educational purposes only and is not recommended as a means of diagnosing or treating an illness. All matters concerning physical and mental health should be supervised by a health practitioner knowledgeable in treating that particular condition. Neither the publisher nor the author directly or indirectly dispenses medical advice, nor do they prescribe any remedies or assume any responsibility for those who choose to treat themselves.

Cataloging-in-Publication data is available from the Library of Congress.

ISBN-13: 978-1-58054-428-3

Printed in the United States of America

Contents

The Healing Aromas of Plants 5

Aroma, The Nose, and The Brain 5

The Essence of the Inner Life of Plants 6

History of Aromatherapy 7

Modern Pioneers of Aromatherapy 8

Aromatherapy Today 9

Synthetic Aromatherapy Products 10

Application of Essential Oils 10

Simple Ways to Use Aromatherapy 11

Extracting Essential Oils 13

Purity of Essential Oils 14

Carrier Oils 14

Blending the Oils 14

Safety with Essential Oils 15

Aromatherapy Research 15

Popular Essential Oils and Their Uses 16

Aromatherapy Treatments 19

Conclusion 21

References 23

Aromatherapy can be defined as the controlled use of essential oils to maintain and promote physical, psychological, and spiritual well-being.

—Gabriel Mojay

The Healing Aromas of Plants

Aromatherapy is the practice of using essential oils derived from botanical sources to treat various physical and emotional illnesses. Due to aromatherapy's therapeutic properties and healing power, people are increasingly using it to improve their lives, and the traditional medical world has taken notice. Scientific research is being conducted around the world to study the therapeutic benefits of essential oils, and the results of numerous studies are promising.

Aroma, The Nose, and The Brain

The reticular system of the brain stem senses and analyzes aromas that enter the body through the nose and mouth. Because aromatic molecules travel directly to that part of the brain, without intermediary processing like some of the other senses, our memories, our emotions, and our present awareness are all interwoven in complex interactions that have biochemical effects on our nervous system and other parts of our body. Herein lies aromatherapy's great ability to heal and bring balance to the mind and body.

The hypothalamus is the part of the brain that oversees the functioning of the endocrine system, which controls hormonal secretion and regulation throughout the body. When triggered by a particular aroma, the hypothalamus becomes stimulated, which in turn affects the pituitary gland and causes a hormonal chain reaction throughout the body that affects emotions and behavior. Hormones also control most cells and organ systems in the body, including the immune system.

Smell is our most sensitive sense; it has the ability to detect only a couple of molecules of a particular aroma and can differentiate between thousands of different scents and aromas. The power of our sense of smell and the cascade of physiological events that it triggers form the foundation of aromatherapy, a unique and fascinating area in the healing arts. Aromas from the essential oils derived from numerous plants can strengthen the immune system, reduce pain, increase energy, relieve stress, and promote an overall feeling of well-being.

> **Fragrant Factoid**
>
> The olfactory cells in your nose are the only place in your entire body where the central nervous system comes in direct contact with the external environment.

The Essence of the Inner Life of Plants

Essential oils are highly concentrated natural substances that are derived from the bark, petals, leaves, resins, and rinds of plants. These plant essences are extracted by various methods, including pressing, distillation, tapping, and heat separation. Most essential oils are colorless, but some, such as cinnamon, have color.

In the Vocabulary of Natural Materials (ISO/D1S9235.2), the International Organization for Standardization (ISO) offers the following definition: "An essential oil is a product made by distillation with either water or steam or by mechanical processing of citrus rinds or by dry distillation of natural materials. Following the distillation, the essential oil is physically separated from the water phase."

Essential oils are not actually oily, but are more similar in substance to water. They evaporate easily when exposed to air, but do not dissolve in water. For this reason, essential oils need to be kept in sealed, colored-glass containers to protect them from air and light.

History of Aromatherapy

The early Egyptians used myrrh, frankincense, cedarwood, coriander, cypress, assai, and juniper oils for mummification and for religious rituals—demonstrating the first recorded use of aromatherapy. They used oils to honor their leaders, pharaohs, and priests. Royalty and the wealthy of ancient Egypt used essential oils as well.

In India, practitioners of ayurvedic medicine utilized essential oils in practicing their healing arts, and scent was an important part of their spiritual lives. Many ancient ayurvedic texts suggest the medicinal use of essential oils, including coriander, ginger, myrrh, sandalwood, and rose.

The Hebrews used essential oils for special purification rituals. After sojourning in Egypt, the Hebrews brought the tradition of essential oils with them to Israel. Spikenard, saffron, cinnamon, frankincense, myrrh, aloe, lily, and camphor are all mentioned in the Song of Solomon in the Hebrew Bible. Certain oils were reserved for sacred rites and forbidden for individual use. In the New Testament, the Gospel of John relates a story in which Mary anointed the feet of Christ with spikenard, filling the room with the ointment's aroma.

The Ancient Greeks considered aromatic plants and oils to be a gift from the gods that had significant spiritual value and power. The Greeks most likely learned the secrets of aromatherapy from the Egyptians. Hippocrates, the father of medicine, recommended scented daily baths and massages with essential oils to promote longevity.

The Romans, who acquired their knowledge of aromatherapy from the Greeks, added scented oils and perfumes to their famous baths, which were an important part of their culture. In addition to the public baths, the Romans used fragrant oils in their homes.

Avicenna, the famous Arabian doctor of the tenth century, was the first to use the process of distillation to create essential oils, although some claim that the Egyptians had also practiced a primitive form of distillation. This was an important development because of the value of essential oils in trade and commerce.

Early Europeans learned of aromatherapy from crusaders returning from the Holy Land, marking the beginning of the French perfume industry. The first charter granted to a French *perfumerie* was given in 1190. Throughout the Middle Ages, bags of strong-smelling herbs were carried or worn by people to protect themselves from demons and disease. During the years of the plague and other life-threatening ailments, distilled aromatics were highly prized and were used as antiseptics to protect and heal.

Fragrant Factoid

The oldest medical text in existence describes a medical practice that relied on aromatic compounds. It was recorded on two clay tablets during the Sumerian period, around 3500 BC.

Modern Pioneers of Aromatherapy
René-Maurice Gattefossé

René-Maurice Gattefossé, a French cosmetic chemist, is one of the most prominent figures in the history of aromatherapy. Gattefossé coined the term *aromatherapie* and around 1936 introduced the theory that essential oils are beneficial for the skin. Gattefossé spent over fifty years studying essential oils and came to realize that they were effective in fighting infections.

Gattefossé was in the process of blending a combination of essential oils for a new perfume when an explosion occurred, burning his arm. He hurried to find the nearest cool liquid in which to plunge his scalded arm. It happened to be a bowl of lavender oil. Gattefossé was amazed by how quickly and effectively the lavender oil relieved his pain. This led him to study the remarkable qualities of healing oils and write prolifically about aromatherapy and its therapeutic properties.

Maurice Godissart

A colleague of Gattefossé's, Maurice Godissart, later opened an aromatherapy clinic in the United States and treated skin cancer, gangrene, osteomalacia, and facial ulcers with lavender oil. Godissart had much success in healing his patients' skin conditions.

Paolo Rovesti

Paolo Rovesti of Milan University in Italy was one of the first scientists to study the effects of essential oils on the mind. In a clinical study, Rovesti administered the fragrances of specific essential oils to patients and found that this therapy served either as a nerve stimulant or as a nerve sedative to treat depression and anxiety.

Marguerite Maury

A prominent French biochemist in the mid–twentieth century, Marguerite Maury believed that the external use of essential oils through massage was the best method of administering them for therapeutic effect. Maury focused on using oils blended for each individual patient depending on their symptoms and disposition. She conducted the bulk of her research in England during the 1950s and developed numerous new aromatherapeutic compounds.

> **Fragrant Factoid**
>
> Rosemary, mugwort, and St. John's wort have long been associated with magic and clairvoyant powers and have been used as magical talismans to fight evil.

Aromatherapy Today

As people look for alternative ways to treat their physical and mental health conditions, some are finding help in the therapeutic properties of aromatherapy.

In an article published in *USA Today,* Dr. Robert Henkin of the Taste and Smell Clinic in Washington, DC, said that aromatherapy is blossoming today because "people are becoming more aware . . . that natural things have natural consequences." He said that aromatherapy is already present in our daily lives—in scented soaps, bath oils, herbs and spices, perfumes, and deodorants. The quantity of essential oils sold in the United States increased by 102.6 million ounces from 2000–2002, according to the Fragrance Materials Association. Sales are up eighteen million dollars over that period.

Synthetic Aromatherapy Products

Because aromatherapy is becoming so popular, manufacturers are now making synthetic copies of essential oils. These scents, however, are not as effective as the natural substances that the practice of aromatherapy is based on. The synthetics do not contain the life force of the plant and cannot produce the same therapeutic results as true essential oils. The actual structure of a plant cannot be duplicated, and the synthetic versions are considered relatively harmless but ineffective.

Application of Essential Oils

Everyone can benefit from the use of essential oils. Whether you inhale peppermint oil each afternoon for a quick energy boost, or relax in a soothing tub with lavender oil before bed, essential oils can be used throughout the day to help reduce stress and increase energy.

Essential oils are usually applied by massage to allow the therapeutic essence to penetrate the skin. The oils affect different areas of the body through the blood and body fluids. Massage is an important part of the process because it helps to increase the essential oil's rate of absorption.

Another form of administration is inhalation, which transports molecules of the essential oil to the lungs and throughout the body. Drops of oil can be added to a humidifier or sprayed in the air. A few drops can be put on a cotton pad and inhaled during the day. Inhaling the oils can have a profound effect on both the body and the mind.

Fragrant Factoid

In Eastern healing, the base chakra is associated with patchouli, frankincense, vetiver, elemi, and myrrh.

The heart chakra is associated with melissa, bergamot, jasmine, rose, and inula.

Simple Ways to Use Aromatherapy

Before using any essential oils, please read the safety information on each individual oil you plan to use. Many oils should not be used in areas where children and pets can come in contact with them.

Bath: Add five to seven drops of essential oil to one ounce of carrier oil. Add this blend to your bath water and mix well before getting into the tub.

Insect repellent: Many essential oils including citronella, peppermint, and lavender act as a natural insect repellent. Sprinkle a few drops of essential oil onto cotton balls or tissues and place near doorways and windows to repel insects.

Easy inhalation: Place three to four drops of essential oil on a tissue. Place the tissue near your nose and inhale. When trying an oil for the first time, use only one drop to ensure that you don't have a sensitivity or reaction to the oil.

Household freshening: Add a few drops of oil to your trash can, laundry, vacuum cleaner bag, drain, or on a tissue in your drawers.

Massage: Add up to twenty drops of essential oil to one ounce of carrier oil such as sweet almond oil and massage onto your skin or your partner's skin. Keep away from the eyes and genitals. Never apply essential oils directly to the skin without first diluting them.

Steam inhalation: Boil two cups of water. Pour the water into a bowl and add three to seven drops of oil. Use fewer drops if you are using an oil that may cause irritation to your mucous membranes (e.g., cinnamon, eucalyptus, rosemary, pine, thyme, cajeput). Place your nose about twelve inches away from the bowl and inhale. Don't inhale the steam constantly, and if you notice any irritation or discomfort stop immediately. Steam inhalation can help with colds and influenza. Energizing oils can be used during the day, and soothing, relaxing oils can be used at night.

Room freshening: Use the steam inhalation method noted above but don't inhale directly. Use up to ten drops of oil. Use fewer drops if you are using an oil that may cause sensitization. Other methods include using an aromatherapy diffuser or lamp scent ring.

Body lotion: Add fifty to sixty drops of essential oil to sixteen ounces of unscented body lotion and mix thoroughly.

Body mist: Add ten to fifteen drops of essential oil to a one-ounce glass misting bottle filled with spring water.

Body oil: Add about twelve to fifteen drops of essential oil to one ounce of carrier oil, such as jojoba or sweet almond oil, and mix well to blend.

Compress: Mix three to five drops of essential oil in a bowl of water. Soak a washcloth in the fragrant water, wring, and apply.

Liniment: Add fifteen to twenty drops of essential oil to one ounce of carrier oil, such as jojoba oil. Shake well to blend.

Liquid soap: Add about thirty to fifty drops of essential oil to eight ounces of unscented liquid hand soap.

Shampoo/conditioner: Add twelve to fifteen drops of essential oil to one ounce of unscented or mild shampoo and mix.

Fragrant Factoid

Among the mystical Sufis, the experience of the divine is closely associated with the rose.

Extracting Essential Oils

The plants used in aromatherapy are cultivated and harvested when they are at their peak of quality. The oil extraction is usually done as soon as possible after harvest to ensure freshness and purity.

Steam Distillation

Steam distillation is the method most frequently used to extract essential oils, and is the most efficient method of extraction for most plants. In distillation, the plant is placed on a mesh sheet in a large copper or stainless steel vat. The plants are usually fresh, but dried plants are sometimes used. Pressurized steam passes through the plant material forcing the oil in the plant to be released. The temperature must be hot enough to release the oil but not so hot as to burn the oil or destroy the plant. The essential oils evaporate with the steam and travel through a tube to the condensation chamber. The oils then form a film that is easily separated from the water and collected in a flask. The essential oils of lavender, geranium, rosemary, clove, cypress, peppermint, sandalwood, and eucalyptus are all extracted by steam distillation.

Cold Pressing

Cold pressing is the most common method of extracting oils from citrus fruits—oranges, limes, grapefruits, lemons, and tangerines. In this process, the fruit is pierced with a sharp object rolling over a trough, releasing the essential oils, which then rise to the surface and separate from the juice.

Enfleurage

Certain delicate flowers are too fragile for steam or cold-press extraction. Instead, a gentler method called enfleurage is used. Enfleurage involves a lengthy process of coating flower petals with an odorless vegetable oil that absorbs the plant's essential oils. Enfleurage typically produces the most concentrated oils.

Solvent Extraction

Solvent extraction is another method to obtain essential oils from delicate plants. In this expensive time-consuming process, the plant is coated with a chemical solvent to extract the essential oils. Rose and jasmine are examples of flowers usually extracted with solvents.

Purity of Essential Oils

Absolutely pure essential oils are required to ensure consistent therapeutic results, so it's critical that you buy products sold by reputable suppliers. An experienced aromatherapist can determine the quality of an essential oil just by smelling it, and they can usually tell synthetic versions and lower quality oils from high-quality natural oils.

Carrier Oils

Pure essential oils should be mixed with a carrier oil before being applied to the skin because the essential oils are highly concentrated and may cause skin irritation. Only a small amount of the essential oil/carrier oil mixture is required for therapeutic results.

Carrier oils should be odorless cold-pressed vegetable oils without additives. Some of the most common carrier oils are sweet almond oil, canola oil, grapeseed oil, sesame oil, jojoba oil, and olive oil. Carrier oils should be refrigerated to retain freshness, and rancid oils should be discarded immediately.

Blending the Oils

Essential oils can be purchased in preblended formulas, and oils can be custom blended to meet individual therapeutic needs. Once one essential oil is combined with another, an entirely new substance is created. So oils that work well together and that create a balanced mixture should be used. For example, a more powerful oil may be combined with a less dominant oil; or a very sweet scent may be blended with a citrus oil to lessen the sweetness. Blending can be a creative experience, and with time, research, and experimentation, you can discover which oils work best together for you.

Safety with Essential Oils

Some essential oils may cause allergic reactions. If you have sensitive skin, you can do a patch test by applying two to three drops of diluted oil to an area on the arm and cover with a bandage. Leave the bandage on overnight and check for a reaction in the morning.

Essential oils are highly concentrated and should be used according to label instructions. Essential oils should only be taken by mouth under the direction of a reputable aromatherapist.

Aromatherapy Research
Weight Loss

A study conducted at Duke University by professor of psychology Susan Schiffman, PhD, used apricot oil to help obese people control their eating. The apricot scent helped the study participants relax and feel less anxious, which is a common reason for overeating. Each person carried a vial of the oil with them and took a sniff when they felt nervous. More than half of the group experienced benefits from the apricot oil.

Memory

In his research, Trygg Engen, a scientist at Brown University, has found a link between memory and essential oils. The olfactory system is connected to the limbic system and memory. In one study, the memory recall process was at least doubled with the addition of scents from the past. A scent that hadn't been experienced for many years brought back memories and images.

Relaxation and Mood Improvement

Susan Schiffman has found beneficial results from using pleasant scents to help women with stress, anxiety, and tension associated with menopause. The scents seem to help release negative emotions and promote positive feelings.

Memorial Sloan-Kettering Cancer Center in New York City is using aromatherapy to help promote relaxation and relieve anxiety among patents, their families, and staff. The scent of vanilla is used to relax patients when they undergo anxiety-inducing procedures such as MRIs. The use of fragrances in hospitals has helped to reduce stress and anxiety when tension is the norm.

The British aromatherapist Robert Tisserand has researched how different scents affect human brain waves. When exposed to stimulating aromas such as black pepper and rosemary, beta brain waves increase. Alpha and theta brain waves increased when rose, lavender, and jasmine were used, resulting in relaxation.

Popular Essential Oils and Their Uses

Basil oil helps to clear and expel mucus, reduce fever, improve circulation, relieve menstrual cramps, and stimulate menstrual flow. It also helps to fight infection and can help relieve depression.

Bergamot oil can help relax muscles and reduce pain. It can also help to fight infections, expel mucus, and promote relaxation, as well as aid indigestion. Oil of bergamot also encourages the growth of new skin tissue.

Cedarwood oil can help ease coughs and reduce the discomforts of colds and flu. Cedarwood oil also promotes urination, functions as an antiseptic to help wounds heal and prevent infection, and helps to ease the pain of arthritis.

Chamomile oil has a refreshing aroma. It is used as a general tonic to soothe the body and mind, and it contains anti-inflammatory properties to help reduce inflammation. It helps to heal skin conditions such as psoriasis, eczema, and sunburn. Oil of chamomile has also been used to ease the pain from arthritis, headaches, and migraines.

Cinnamon oil stimulates and warms the body. It can be mixed with a carrier oil and used in massage to warm the skin.

Clary sage oil helps to calm the nervous system and relieve depression. It helps to balance the emotions and is a nervous system tonic. It also helps to relieve muscle pain and spasm.

Cypress oil can calm the nervous system and relieve stress. It also helps with pain and muscle aches.

Eucalyptus oil can be used to treat colds, allergies, coughs, flu, sinusitis, sore throats, and tonsillitis. It is also considered beneficial in helping to alleviate the pain of a sore throat. Eucalyptus oil helps to fight infections, whether viral or bacterial.

Fennel oil helps to rid the body of toxins. It is also used to help control the appetite to aid with weight loss and is sometimes recommended for urinary tract infections. It is also used for irregular menstrual cycles, PMS, fluid retention, and the symptoms of menopause.

Geranium oil helps with diarrhea, gallstones, and urinary tract infections. It is also recommended to treat sore throats and tonsillitis.

Ginger oil is commonly used for gastrointestinal disorders. It also helps to increase immunity and protect the body from illness.

Jasmine oil relieves coughs and gynecological problems. It can be massaged into the lower back to ease the pain from menstrual cramps and induce menstrual flow. Jasmine oil is often recommended to soothe the discomforts of menopause. It has also been used to help ease the pain of childbirth.

Juniper oil helps to reduce pain and muscle aches. It increases urination and can stimulate menstrual flow. It can fight infection and water retention.

Lavender oil is a versatile oil used for many conditions, including promoting restful sleep. It can be used for digestive problems, respiratory disorders, pain and muscle aches, skin disorders, and wounds. It should be used only in small quantities because of its strength.

Lemon oil is used for respiratory disorders such as bronchitis, coughs, sore throats, flu and cold symptoms. It contains antibacterial properties. It aids in digestion and strengthens the immune system.

Myrrh has been used for thousands of years. It helps to boost the immune system and fight infections. It helps with digestion and stimulates the appetite. Some aromatherapists recommend myrrh for respiratory complaints, fungal infections, healing wounds, menstrual complaints, and skin disorders.

Orange oil helps relieve tension and relax the body. It is used for respiratory problems such as bronchitis, colds. and flu. It increases immunity to strengthen the entire body. It is also used to aid digestion, nervous disorders, diarrhea, obesity, and muscle and joint aches.

Peppermint oil is used in cases of fever and headache and to increase energy levels. It stimulates the nervous system to increase energy and reduce fatigue and also helps with digestion and nausea. Peppermint oil relaxes muscle tension, relieves headaches and migraines, and helps with some skin conditions.

Rose oil is probably the most expensive of the essential oils. It takes approximately one hundred pounds of rose petals to extract 0.5 ounces of oil. Aromatherapists recommend rose oil for digestion, coughs, wound healing, congestion, hormonal balance, skin conditions, headaches, and inflammation.

Rosemary oil is taken from the flowering tops of the plant. It is used for digestion, arthritis, coughs, depression, scalp problems, relaxation, headaches, muscle pain, cardiovascular disorders, respiratory conditions, memory, and circulation.

Rosewood oil helps to calm the nervous system and helps to ease depression, anxiety, and stress. It fights infection, increases immunity, relieves pain, and can stimulate sexual desire.

Spearmint oil helps stomach problems and can aid digestion and help relieve nausea.

Tea tree oil is well known for its antiseptic properties, and can help fight viral, bacterial, and fungal infections. It is used to treat acne, burns, cuts, dandruff, respiratory ailments, coughs, urinary tract infections, candida, and eczema.

Thyme oil helps to increase immunity and prevent infections. It is used for respiratory conditions such as asthma, bronchitis, tonsillitis, coughs, colds, sinusitis, and sore throats.

Aromatherapy Treatments

Abrasions, cuts, and wounds: Clean the affected area. Apply a few drops of lavender oil or tea tree oil to the area. Cover with a bandage. Reapply the oil two to three times a day until the area has healed.

Athlete's foot: Mix together two drops of lavender oil and one drop of tea tree oil. Use a cotton swab to apply to the feet and in between the toes. The feet can also be soaked in a foot bath with ten drops of tea tree oil. Soak for about fifteen minutes.

Burns: Lavender oil or tea tree oil can be applied to a burn to soothe and promote healing.

Calming: Add to a bath four drops chamomile oil, two drops clary sage oil, and two drops of orange oil.

Common cold: Combine three drops of lemon oil and one drop of myrrh. Add to a hot bath, relax, and inhale.

Cough: Blend three drops of eucalyptus oil, two drops of thyme oil, and four drops of pine oil with four teaspoons of carrier oil. Massage this blend into the chest area.

Depression: Add two drops chamomile oil, three drops lavender oil, and two drops clary sage oil to a bath. Relax and breathe deeply.

Headache: Mix three drops lavender oil, two drops peppermint oil, and two drops carrier oil. Massage this blend into the temples.

Hyperactivity: For children, add one drop of chamomile oil and one drop of lavender oil to a bath. Let the child soak for a few minutes. For adults, a blend for the bath could include three drops lavender oil, two drops basil oil, two drops fennel oil, and two drops chamomile oil.

Insect bites/bee stings: Chamomile oil can be applied to the area a few times a day to relieve pain, itching, and swelling. A combination of one ounce carrier oil, four drops pine oil, four drops tea tree oil, three drops eucalyptus oil, and one drop peppermint oil can also be used. This combination also works as an insect repellent.

Insomnia: Add four drops chamomile oil, three drops valerian oil, and one drop basil oil to a warm bath and breathe deeply.

Menstrual pain and cramps: Blend together eight drops peppermint oil, five drops lavender oil, five drops cypress oil and two tablespoons carrier oil. Massage into the lower back, abdomen, and shoulders. Take a few minutes to relax.

Muscle aches and pains: For exercise-induced aches and pains, try four drops basil oil, four drops rosemary oil, three drops peppermint oil, and two drops of ginger oil. Blend with one ounce of carrier oil. Massage into the affected areas.

PMS: Add a few drops of any combination of the following to a warm bath: bergamot, chamomile, clary sage, geranium, juniper, and jonquil. A massage oil for PMS could include three ounces carrier oil, eight drops chamomile oil, eight drops clary sage oil, four drops fennel oil, three drops geranium oil, and three drops ylang-ylang oil.

Sinus problems: Blend two drops rosemary oil, one drop geranium oil and one drop eucalyptus oil; place on a cotton ball and breathe deeply.

Stress: Mix four drops cypress oil, two drops geranium oil, two drops chamomile oil, and one teaspoon carrier oil. Place on a cotton ball and breathe deeply or massage into the neck and shoulders.

> **Fragrant Factoid**
> In Mexico, a clove of garlic is still hung around the neck of newborns as a protection against sickness and evil spirits.

Conclusion

As we learn to be more sensitive to smells and the way they influence us, we will be able to determine how to best use essential oils. As the previous list suggests, the effects of aromatherapy are wide-reaching. The use of essential oils as part of a natural health routine could lead to an improved state of health for men, women and children alike.

References

"Aromatherapy 101: What Is Aromatherapy?" http://wlnaturalhealth.com/aromatherapy-articles/what-is-aromatherapy.htm.

Barson, Andy. "Amateur Aromatherapy," http://andybarson.co.uk/Aroma/frames.htm.

Battaglia, S. *The Complete Guide to Aromatherapy.* Virginia, Queensland, Australia: The Perfect Potion Ltd., 1997.

Belaiche, P. *Traite de phytotherapie et d'aromathérapie.* Vols. 1–3. Paris: Maloine, 1979.

Berwick, Ann. *Holistic Aromatherapy.* St. Paul, MN: Llewellyn Publications, 1994, 5.

Bienfang, Ralph. *The Subtle Sense, Key to the World of Odors.* Oklahoma City; University of Oklahoma Press, 1946.

Blumenthal, M., Busse, W. R., et al. *The Complete German Commission E Monographs: Therapeutic Guide to Herbal Medicines.* Austin, TX : American Botanical Council; Boston, MA: Integrative Medicine Communication, 1998.

Buchbauer, G. *New Results in Aromatherapy Research.* 24th International Symposium on Essential Oils. July 21–24, 1993. Berlin, Germany: Technical University.

Buckle, J. *Clinical Aromatherapy in Nursing.* London, U.K.: Arnold, 1997.

Castleman, Michael. *Nature's Cures.* Emmaus, Pennsylvania: Rodale, 1996, 32.

"Essential Oil Uses," http://www.aromaweb.com/articles/uses.asp.

Fuchs, N., Jager, W., et al. "Systemic absorption of topically applied carvone: influence of massage technique." *J Soc Cosmet Chem.* 1997; 48(6): 277–82.

Gattefossé, M. *Gattefossé's Aromatherapy* [*Aromathérapie: les huiles essentielles hormones végétales*]. Tisserand, R., editor. Davies, L., translator. Saffron Walden, U.K.: C.W. Daniel Co. Ltd., 1993.

Hainer, Cathy. *USA Today.* "Aromatherapy wafts into mainstream science business," July 1, 1992.

http://wellseo.com/aromatherapy/facts.php?PHPSESSID=202fea67d42218f61164fcfdf82e5c02

http://wlnaturalhealth.com/aromatherapy-articles/what-is-aromatherapy.htm

http://www.naha.org/what_is_an_essential_oil.htm

Jager, W., Buchbauer, G., et al. "Percutaneous absorption of lavender oil from a massage oil." *J Soc Cosmet Chem* 1992; 43 (1): 49–54.

Keville, Kathi. "Your Nose Knows, Aromatherapy Today." *Herbs for Health.*

Lavabre, Marcel F. *Aromatherapy Workbook.* Rochester, VT: Healing Arts Press, 1990.

Lawless, J. *The Encyclopedia of Essential Oils.* Shaftesbury, U.K.: Element, 1992.

Lawless, Julia. *The Illustrated Encyclopedia of Essential Oils.* Rockport, MA: Element Books, Inc., 1995.

Manniche, Lise. *Sacred Luxuries: Fragrance, Aromatherapy & Cosmetics in Ancient Egypt.* Ithaca, NY: Cornell University Press, 1999.

Maxwell-Hudson, Clare. *Aromatherapy Massage.* New York: DK Publishing, 1996.

Mills, S. *Out of the Earth.* London: Viking Arkana, 1991, 338.

Paltz, J. *Le Fascinant Pouvoir des Huiles Essentielles.* Publisher unknown, 1984.

Price, S., Price, L. *Aromatherapy for Health Professionals.* London: Churchill Livingstone, 1995.

Reader's Digest Family Guide to Natural Medicine. Pleasantville, NY: Reader's Digest Association, Inc., 1993, 328.

Tisserand, R., Balacs, T. *Essential Oil Safety.* London: Churchill Livingstone, 1996.

Tisserand, Robert B. *The Art of Aromatherapy.* Rochester, VT: Healing Arts Press, 1977.

"Top Ten Essential Oils," http://www.naha.org/top_10.htm

Valnet, J. *The Practice of Aromatherapy.* Rochester, VT: Healing Arts Press, 1990.

Vukovic, Laurel. "Breathe Deeply . . . and Relax." *Natural Health,* Nov–Dec 1995, 64.

Wilder, Louise Beebe. *The Fragrant Path.* New York, NY: Macmillan Company, 1932.

Wilson, Roberta. *A Complete Guide to Understanding and Using Aromatherapy.* Garden City, NY: Doubleday, 1995, 5.

Wilson, Roberts. *Aromatherapy for Vibrant Health and Beauty.* Berkeley, California: North Atlantic Books, 1992.

Worwood, Valerie Ann. *The Complete Book of Essential Oils and Aromatherapy.* New York: Avery Publishing Group, 1995.

Wren, R.C. *Potter's New Cyclopaedia of Botanical Drugs and Preparations.* Saffron Walden, U.K.: C.S. Daniel, 1998.